Type 1 Diabetes

How to Easily Treat and Manage Type 1 Diabetes

Hillary A. Charles

Table of Contents

INTRODUCTION

There are problems, you can push away or avoid the brief- and long-term problems. Controlling your blood sugar levels will help you control the symptoms and stop further damage.

Diabetes complications are related to poor blood sugar control, and that means you must work carefully with your physician and diabetes team to properly manage your bloodstream sugars (or your child's bloodstream sugar).

Diabetes is a significant disease. Pursuing your diabetes treatment solution takes round-the-clock dedication. But your attempts are advantageous. Careful diabetes treatment can lessen your threat of serious - even life-threatening - problems.

This guide will help you maximize your insulin sensitivity, attain your ideal body weight, improve your digestive health, gain energy, live an active life, and feel the best you've felt in years.

CHAPTER 1

Can type 2 diabetes become type 1?

It isn't easy for type 2 diabetes to carefully turn into type 1 diabetes.

However, Type 2 diabetes is the most typical type, type 1 diabetes frequently develops whenever a person is more youthful, although it may appear in folks of any age.

Misdiagnosis

It's possible for a person with type 1 diabetes to get an incorrect analysis of type 2 diabetes if the medical diagnosis occurs in adulthood. This example may become more likely to happen if the individual is also obese or has other risk factors for type 2 diabetes, like a sedentary lifestyle. Though it is uncommon,

Instead, to diagnose diabetes, a health care provider will

perform several blood sugar assessments. However, the results won't allow these to differentiate between your two types.

They could also perform blood tests to check on for antibodies that attack insulin-secreting beta cells in the pancreas. The existence of the antibodies results in a person has type 1 diabetes. 90% of patients with type 1 diabetes are located to have these antibodies. Another test that helps determine whether one has type 1 or type 2 diabetes is a C-peptide test.

Type 1 vs. type 2 diabetes

Although they cause comparable symptoms, generally, to create juvenile diabetes, Type 1 diabetes can be an autoimmune disease, changes in lifestyle will not invert type 1 diabetes, however they can help with blood sugar control and could reduce the threat of health-related complications.

With those who find themselves 45 years or older having an increased potential for developing this problem.

However, it's important to notice that age is not really a reliable diagnostic tool for the kind of diabetes a person has. Given that weight problems is so common among people of all age groups, type 2 diabetes may appear as soon as childhood.

This sort of diabetes inhibits your body's ability to create and use insulin. And weight problems, can boost the probability of developing type 2 diabetes.

Some individuals can control the symptoms of type 2 diabetes by causing changes in lifestyle. These can include doing about 150 minutes of light-to-moderate exercise weekly, slimming down, and eating a healthy, balanced diet.

People with more complex type 2 diabetes may need to take medications, to aid blood sugar control.

Much like other autoimmune disorders, analysts don't realize what can cause type 1 diabetes, for example, like a viral illness,

Once type 1 diabetes is rolling out, these beta cells are crucial for producing insulin, so people who have type 1 diabetes cannot get this to hormone.

Both hereditary and environmental factors also are likely involved in type 2 diabetes. However, type 2 diabetes has nearer links to lifestyle options and diet.

Some individuals with type 2 diabetes should inject insulin to control their blood sugar. However, it is possible to control this problem without insulin.

Insulin dependency

People who have type 1 diabetes might need to make changes in lifestyle alone, however, won't prevent or invert type 1 diabetes.

Because of this, people who have type 1 diabetes are

reliant on insulin, and the problem may also be called insulin-dependent diabetes.

Despite having regular monitoring and regular insulin shots or the utilization of the insulin pump, they could develop dangerously high blood sugar levels sometimes.

When blood glucose spikes occur, they could need further insulin or crisis medical care.

People who have type 2 diabetes will require insulin if other treatments are inadequate in assisting them manage their blood sugar levels. They could also need insulin if there are contraindications to non-insulin diabetes medications, or if the problem, which is usually intensifying, becomes chronic with significant decrease in pancreas capability to create insulin. However, insulin enable you to treat either type.

Many people with type 2 also utilize it is in more complex stages of the problem or if other treatments aren't successful.

And they might not cause symptoms whatsoever. However, sometimes life-threatening problems.

The first symptoms of diabetes might include increased thirst, increased daytime and night-time urination, and unexplained weight reduction.

particularly if one has a family background of diabetes.

CHAPTER 2

Type 1 Diabetes Symptoms

However, the symptoms may appear suddenly. In the event that you observe that you or your son or daughter have many of the symptoms the following, make a scheduled appointment to start to see the doctor.

And your body loses its capability to make insulin. However, at that time, there's still insulin in the torso so sugar levels remain normal.

As time passes, a decreasing amount of insulin is manufactured in the torso, but that may take years. When you forget about insulin in the torso, blood sugar levels rise quickly, and these symptoms can quickly develop:

- Extreme weakness and/or tiredness

- Extreme thirst-dehydration

- Increased urination

- Abdominal pain

- Nausea and/or vomiting

- Blurry vision

- Wounds that don't heal well

- Irritability or quick feeling changes

- Changes to (or lack of) menstruation

Indicators will vary from symptoms for the reason that they could be assessed objectively; Indications of type 1 diabetes include:

- Weight loss-despite consuming more

- Rapid heartrate

- Reduced blood circulation pressure (dropping below 90/60)

- Lower body temperature (below 97° F)

There can be an overall insufficient public knowing of the signs or symptoms of type 1 diabetes. Making yourself alert to the signs or symptoms of type 1 diabetes is a superb way to be proactive about your wellbeing and the fitness of your family users. In the event that you notice these indicators, it's possible you have (or your son or daughter has) type 1 diabetes. A health care provider can make that analysis by checking blood sugar levels.

CHAPTER 3

Type 1 Diabetes Causes

It isn't completely clear what causes type 1 diabetes. Experts can say for certain that genes are likely involved; there can be an inherited susceptibility. Something must trip the disease fighting capability, causing it to carefully turn against itself and resulting in type 1 diabetes.

Genes Are likely involved in Type 1 Diabetes

Some individuals cannot develop type 1 diabetes; that's because they don't have the hereditary coding that research workers have associated with type 1 diabetes. Researchers have determined that type 1 diabetes can form in individuals who have a specific HLA complicated. HLA means human being leukocyte antigen, and antigens function is to cause an immune system response in the torso. And all are on chromosome 6.

Such as arthritis rheumatoid, ankylosing spondylitis, or juvenile arthritis rheumatoid.

What Can Result in Type 1 Diabetes

Here's the complete process of what goes on with a viral contamination: Whenever a computer virus invades your body, the disease fighting capability starts to create antibodies that battle chlamydia. T cells are responsible for making the antibodies, and they also assist in fighting the computer virus.

However, the T cell products (antibodies) can eliminate the beta cells, as soon as all the beta cells within you have been damaged,

But that original viral contamination is what's thought to result in the introduction of type 1 diabetes.

Don't assume all virus can cause the T cells to carefully

turn against the beta cells. The disease will need to have antigens that are similar enough to the antigens in beta cells, and the ones viruses include:

- B4 strain of the coxsackie B virus (which can result in a selection of illnesses from gastrointestinal problems to myocarditis-inflammation of the muscle area of the heart)

- German measles

- Mumps

- Rotavirus (which generally causes diarrhea)

Analysts don't all acknowledge this, however, many think that the protein in cow's dairy act like a proteins that settings T cell creation called glycodelin1.

Research workers have made significant improvement in understanding the reason for type 1 diabetes, the medical community desires to raised understand the instances of diabetes to be able to avoid it.

CHAPTER 4

Type 1 Diabetes Risk Factors

That hereditary marker is situated on chromosome 6, you might develop type 1. (However, getting the necessary HLA complicated is not really a guarantee that you'll develop diabetes; in truth, significantly less than 10% of individuals with the "right" organic(es) actually develop type 1.)

Other risk factors for type 1 diabetes include:

Viral infections: Experts have discovered that certain infections may trigger the introduction of type 1 diabetes by leading to the disease fighting capability to carefully turn against the body-instead of helping it combat infection and sickness. Infections that are thought to result in type 1 include: German measles, coxsackie, and mumps.

In America, Chinese language people have a lesser threat of developing type 1,

Geography: It appears that individuals who reside in north climates are in an increased risk for developing type 1 diabetes. It's been recommended that individuals who reside in north countries are indoors more (especially in the wintertime), and which means that they're in nearer closeness to each other-potentially resulting in more viral attacks.

Conversely, experts have pointed out that more instances are diagnosed in the wintertime in north countries; the medical diagnosis rate falls in the summertime.

If a member of family has (or had) type 1, the probability of the youngster developing type 1 is greater than if just one single mother or father has (or had) diabetes. Analysts have pointed out that if the daddy has type 1,

Type 1 diabetes can be an autoimmune condition since it causes the body's disease fighting capability to carefully turn against itself. and for that reason, having one particular disorder could make you much more likely to build up type 1.

CHAPTER 5

Type 1 Diabetes Problems

There are problems, you can push away or avoid the brief- and long-term problems. Controlling your blood sugar levels will help you control the symptoms and stop further damage.

Diabetes complications are related to poor blood sugar control, and that means you must work carefully with your physician and diabetes team to properly manage your bloodstream sugars (or your child's bloodstream sugar).

Short-term Diabetes Complications

Hypoglycemia: Hypoglycemia is low blood sugar (blood glucose). For example, decreases the blood sugar level invest a dose greater than 81mg) and alcoholic beverages (alcohol retains the liver organ from releasing blood sugar).

You will find three degrees of hypoglycemia, and severe. you'll be able to prevent a lot of more serious problems; Very hardly ever).

The signs or symptoms of low blood sugar are usually easy to identify:

- Rapid heartbeat

- Sweating

- Paleness of skin

- Anxiety

- Numbness in fingertips, feet, and lips

- Sleepiness

- Confusion

- Headache

- Slurred speech

Without blood sugar to fuel the body, it begins to use body fat to get its energy.

When fat is divided by your body, ketones are released. When way too many ketones build-up in the bloodstream, it creates the bloodstream acidic, resulting in diabetic ketoacidosis if the problem isn't handled.

The signs or symptoms of DKA are:

- Frequent urination

- Extreme thirstiness

- Abdominal pain

- Weight loss

- Fruity smell on breathing (that's the smell of ketones released from the body)

- Cold skin

- Confusion

- Weakness

If you believe you (or your son or daughter) has DKA, you can easily confirm it with two at-home exams:

You have high bloodstream sugar (blood sugar),

You can immediately test. You may get ketone strips at your neighborhood pharmacy; The remove will change a deep crimson if way too many ketones are in the torso. (If you can't urinate, you should then have the ability to urinate.)

Diabetic ketoacidosis must be treated, in order as soon as you confirm DKA, call your physician. In the event that you don't have any ketone strips available but nonetheless suspect DKA, go directly to the nearest medical center er immediately to be examined.

Long-term Diabetes Complications

By firmly controlling your blood sugar level (or your child's blood sugar level), you can avoid long-term problems of type 1 diabetes. Essentially, if you work to steer clear of the short-term problems, you'll also be doing some long-range planning and preventing the problems outlined in this section.

Uncontrolled blood sugar can, as time passes, harm the body's small and large arteries.

Harm to your tiny arteries causes microvascular problems;

Microvascular Complications: Eye, Kidney, and Nerve Disease

You have small arteries that may be damaged by poor blood sugar control. Damaged arteries don't deliver bloodstream as well as they ought to, so leading to other problems,

Eyes: Due to type 1 diabetes, or harm to the retina,

Kidneys: If untreated, kidney disease (also known as diabetic nephropathy) leads to dialysis and/or kidney transplant. Uncontrolled (or badly handled) diabetes will probably eventually cause the kidneys to fail; they'll struggle to clean the bloodstream like they need to. To avoid diabetic nephropathy, you (or your son or daughter) should be examined each year for microalbuminuria, which really is a condition that's an early on indication of kidney problems. The test steps how much proteins are within the urine. When the kidneys start to have problems, they begin to release too much proteins.

Nerves: Nerve harm caused by diabetes is also called diabetic neuropathy. The small arteries "give food to" your nerves, then your nerves will eventually be broken as well.

Autonomic, proximal, diabetic peripheral neuropathy is the most typical form of nerve harm, and it frequently impacts the nerves heading to your toes. They could also experience pain,

The sore may become infected, chlamydia can spread,

and still left untreated, the feet might need to have surgery to keep carefully the infection from distributing more.

Macrovascular Complications: The Heart

Leading to plaque to eventually build-up and potentially resulting in a coronary attack. To prevent cardiovascular disease consequently of diabetes, however, it's also advisable to make heart-healthy options in the areas you will ever have: don't smoke cigarettes, keep your blood circulation pressure in order, and focus on your cholesterol.

These are the primary problems, by carefully managing your blood sugar, you can prevent these problems.

Type 1 Diabetes Avoidance

Currently, there is absolutely no way to avoid type 1 diabetes. Experts are still trying to fully understand what can cause or sets off type 1; without completely knowing that, it's difficult to avoid the disease.

Which sometimes can be avoided by taking proper care of your body-watching your daily diet and staying toned and active.

With type 1 diabetes, you can push away or avoid the short-term and long-term problems of the condition.

CHAPTER 6

Type 1 Diabetes and Exercise

Staying fit and energetic during your life has benefits, however the biggest one for individuals with diabetes is this: it can help you control diabetes and stop long-term complications.

Exercise helps it be simpler to control your blood sugar (blood sugars) level. Exercise benefits people who have type 1 since it boosts your insulin sensitivity. Quite simply, after exercise, if your son or daughter has type 1 diabetes, For more information about how exactly to safely include exercise into your son or daughter's regular, especially heart disease. people who have diabetes are vulnerable to developing clogged arteries (arteriosclerosis), which can result in a coronary attack.

Exercise helps maintain your center healthy and strong.

Additionally, there are traditional advantages of exercise:

- Lower blood circulation pressure

- Better control of weight

- Leaner, more powerful muscles

- Stronger bones

- More energy

One individual who certainly understands the advantages of exercise in managing type 1 diabetes is Jay Cutler, quarterback for the Chicago Bears. He was identified as having type 1 diabetes in 2008, however the disease hasn't interfered along with his soccer career.

Unless you currently exercise (or if your son or daughter isn't as dynamic as she or he should be), speak to your doctor prior to starting. Particularly if you're a grown-up with type 1 diabetes, you ought to have a complete physical to ensure you're prepared to be more energetic.

Which is specially important if you currently have blocked arteries or high blood circulation pressure. For example. As you start a fitness program, your physician will help you find out the best workout program which allows you to enter form but doesn't drive the body too far.

Before you start exercising, you will need to create realistic goals. In the event that you haven't exercised much lately, you aren't heading to leap into owning a marathon. Actually, you are not even heading to leap into owning a 5k.

Allow yourself a while to develop to a reliable, challenging workout routine.

Finally, you do not want to be hypoglycemic throughout a work-out, so you will have to do some planning.

Several Exercise Suggestions

You can find three main types of exercise-aerobic, weight training, and versatility work. You should try to have a good balance of most three.

- Aerobic Exercises

- Cardio exercises include:

- Walking

- Jogging/Running

- Tennis

- Basketball

- Swimming

- Biking

You should try to reach least thirty minutes of aerobic fitness exercise most times of the week. Actually, the American Diabetes Association suggests 150 minutes of moderate strength aerobic exercise weekly, which computes to thirty minutes five times a week. If you believe that you can't find thirty minutes,

Also, stretch your creativeness as it pertains to fitting in exercise. Go for a walk at lunchtime, or get everyone out after supper for a casino game of basketball.

Strength Training

Strength training offers you trim, efficient muscles, looked after can help you maintain strong, healthy bones.

Weight training exercise is one of the very most used weight training techniques,

If you are starting a weight training exercise program, be sure you learn how to use all the gear.

Weight lifting for 20-30 minutes several times weekly is enough to get the entire advantages of strength training.

If you're struggling to exercise in a fitness center, canned goods or perhaps a 5 lb handbag of flour can be utilized for weight training.

Flexibility Training

With versatility training, extending before and after exercise (especially after exercise) reduces muscle pain and also relaxes muscle tissue.

Stick to Your Fitness Plan

Your long-term health depends upon it, in order tough as it might be to find time or even to motivate you to ultimately exercise, keep being energetic.

One of the better ways to be sure you stick with a fitness plan is to combine it up-and do stuff that you truly enjoy. If there are a sport that you love, try to become a member of a league. If you want running, join races to give a problem and an objective.

Exercise with friends;

Exercise will help you avoid serious long-term problems of diabetes.

CHAPTER 7

Type 1 Diabetes and Insulin

It's essential to take insulin when you yourself have type 1 diabetes. The body can't properly get the power and fuel it requires from glucose. It was previously called insulin-dependent diabetes.

To learn about how exactly the hormone insulin works, you'll be immersed in the wonderful world of insulin, and it could feel overwhelming initially. A couple of dosages to calculate, your diabetes treatment team will there be to help you. They are able to walk you through the fundamentals of insulin dosing.

Types of Insulin

With type 1 diabetes, you'll need to consider insulin on a regular basis, and there are various kinds insulin you may take. And you'll probably take a mixture of insulin.

The types of insulin are:

Rapid-acting: This sort of insulin calls for effect within quarter-hour, and also you take it before meals.

It's also used before meals, but its impact lasts much longer than rapid-acting insulin. It really is injected thirty minutes to one hour before foods.

It's generally used twice each day, To be able to function effectively,

Long-acting: Much like intermediate-acting insulin, long-acting insulin continues for 20-24 hours,

Pre-mixed: A pre-mixed insulin combines two other styles of insulin-for example, a rapid-acting and intermediate-acting insulin. This assures which you have the right amount of insulin to protect the bolus and basal secretions.

Just How Much Insulin Can You Take?

And she or he will continue to work with you to determine the best insulin plan. She or he will take under consideration your weight, age group, diet, general health, and treatment goals.

You will modify the insulin doses, based about how your blood sugar level responds. That you have a certain dosage before breakfast. In case your blood sugar is too much afterward,

Where Can You Inject The Insulin?

You will find four main areas to inject insulin:

- Abdomen

- Back again of Arm

- Thighs

- Hips/Buttocks

Several notes about insulin injection sites:

- Eventually, you should rotate shot sites.

- Inject the insulin under your skin. It might be difficult to provide yourself the shot for the reason that area without assistance,

Newer, Easier Methods to Inject Insulin

You have many choices for "insulin delivery, less unpleasant, and far more convenient methods for getting insulin in to the body.

For a long period, now, many people are employing insulin pens and other shot devices. and could be prolonged to 180 times, therefore you could go for half a year and never have to think about mealtime insulin shots.

Another option for insulin delivery can be an insulin pump. That's a battery-driven device that provides the body insulin, similar to the pancreas will, and it can it constantly. The pump is worn externally (just like a pager or cellular phone, it could be clipped on your belt), but there is generally a pipe and needle that send insulin under your skin.

Be aware of Insulin Reassurance

There are a great number of options and what to think about as it pertains to insulin. However, when you can get a deal with about how insulin works and its own effect on the body.

CHAPTER 8

Type 1 Diabetes Treatments.

And that means you need to take insulin to be able to control your blood glucose to stay healthy and prevent serious complications.

Controlling Glucose in T1D Has but One Treatment-Insulin

The first and primary medication share with someone with T1D is insulin. It has been our standard method of treatment because the finding and following creation of insulin in humans for greater than a century. Both medications approved by the meals and Medication Administration (FDA) to control blood sugar in people who have type 1 diabetes are-insulin and Symlin.

Blood sugar is the primary source of sugars that the body depends upon for gas (instant energy). However, in order for the body to use blood sugar properly, you'll need to get insulin.

Insulin was initially successfully found in humans in 1922. Insulin was made synthetically, or exogenously, indicating that it is currently manufactured in the laboratory.

Understand the Types of Insulin Open to MAINTAIN Good Glucose Control

All sorts of insulin have the same impact in assisting control your bloodstream glucose, and must be injected through your skin therefore the body or inhaled in to the lungs which means that your body can utilize it. If insulin were swallowed, as with a tablet form, your abdomen acids would break it down so that it wouldn't be accessible to get the job done of controlling blood sugar.

Your lifestyle, as well as your overall needs. However, how quickly they take action, and exactly how long they last. First, there are four basic types of insulin:

Rapid-acting insulin starts employed in about a quarter-hour and is maintained between three to four 4 hours.

The purpose of taking insulin is to keep the blood sugar in a wholesome range; this is known as well controlled. You may check your bloodstream sugars and consider the amount of carbs in the next food or snack to be able to look for the amount of insulin you'll need.

Furthermore, to daily blood sugar checks, which really is a blood measure that delivers helpful information to your estimated blood sugar levels over 90 days. Generally speaking, 5%.

Below can be a summary of the types of insulins, if they can be purchased in a vial, which takes a syringe to get ready the shot or an injectable pen where the insulin is premeasured into a tool that is preparing to use.

Treatments for T1D: Beyond Insulin

Pramlintide, brand Symlin, neither is amylin. The product was made to fill up that space. Reduce tummy emptying and decrease the rise in post-meal bloodstream sugars.

It can't be blended with insulin-Note it must be studied separately. It is available by injectable pen only. together with insulin, 8-7.1 units each day.

Furthermore, pramlintide has been proven to achieve an advantageous decrease in A1c of -0.24-0.58% and could support weight lack of 1.8-3.5 pounds. While these benefits are quite appealing, you will have to decide if you are regularly taking yet another 3-5 injections per day. Another factor is medical health insurance reimbursement, that will vary and really should be examined before making a decision whether to include this treatment or not.

Understanding the Restricts of Treatment Plans

Specifically, metformin; however, this agency will stipulate who are able to receive the medication as well as for what conditions. These details is dependent on results of medical trials which have been conducted to observe how well people react to the medication in comparison with no treatment or even to another examined medication.

It is becoming more and more less uncommon for drugs to be recommended for reasons beyond its original approval-a practice called "off-label" use. What which means is that whenever there are no studies to back up its use for a specific patient, your physician might contemplate it worth providing you to try. This happens when the most common or standard treatments aren't working so prescribing a medication that spent some time working for similar conditions is given.

Although it may be safe and good for use these drugs in a fashion that will not fit with the initial FDA approval, in addition, it means that if someone runs on the drug off-label, insurance firms might not cover the price.

Therefore, your degree of exercise level, plus your meals and snack foods (eg, just how many carbs), may also be considered when planning your insulin needs.

This agency will stipulate who are able to receive the medication as well as for what conditions. These details depends on results of scientific trials which have been conducted to observe how well people react to the medication in comparison with no treatment or even to another examined medication. Your physician might contemplate it worth providing you to try.

Although it may be safe and good for use these drugs in a

fashion that will not fit with the initial FDA approval, In addition, it means that if someone runs on the drug off-label, insurance firms might not cover the price.

Type 1 Diabetes Clinical Tests

Different medical trials assist in improving health care and standard of living of individuals with type 1 diabetes (also known as type 1 diabetes mellitus). Some clinical tests evaluate ways to avoid and control this endocrine disease. Other studies seek to judge how type 1 diabetes impacts other body systems, its romantic relationship to other diseases, and improvements in diagnostic and monitoring tools.

CHAPTER 9

Ill Day Management Tips whenever your Child Has Type 1 Diabetes

Having a sick and tired child can be challenging-getting time off work and acquiring a last-minute doctor's appointment isn't always easy. However, when your unwell child also happens to have type 1 diabetes, it presents another set of problems associated with insulin and blood sugar (blood glucose) management. This guide addresses some important factors to bear in mind next time your son or daughter with type 1 diabetes feels under the elements.

Checking Blood Sugar And Ketones

Even the most typical ailments, can cause your son or daughter's blood sugar levels to go up.

Complicating matters, your son or daughter's blood sugar levels could possibly drop too low if she or he is throwing up or has halted eating.

You just cannot be certain how a sickness will affect your son or daughter's blood glucose-that's why it is important to check their levels more regularly than you normally would. An over-all guideline to aim for is to check on their blood sugar every 2-3 hours, your child may necessitate more or fewer inspections, depending on your wellbeing care professional's suggestions.

Furthermore, to check blood sugar levels, in people who have type 1 diabetes, common ailments can result in diabetic ketoacidosis, a disorder seen as an acidic blood triggered by the discharge of way too many ketones.

Ketones are released whenever your body does not have enough insulin, if ketones remain present, that is clearly an indication that your son or daughter needs more insulin.

Insulin Modifications During Ill Days

Oftentimes, your son or daughter might not want or have the ability to eat when ill. However, it's still essential that your son or daughter helps to keep taking insulin when they're unwell. Without insulin, your body will vacation resort to losing fat for energy, which can result in diabetic ketoacidosis.

Because disease can wreak havoc on blood sugar levels, you'll likely need to change your son or daughter's insulin dosage. The amount of adjustment is totally unique to your son or daughter. Plus, the severe nature of the condition and treatments used also element in.

Use your son or daughter's blood sugar levels as helpful information when modifying insulin. When you have any questions about how exactly to adjust your son or daughter's insulin on ill days, call your wellbeing care professional.

Drink and food Guidelines

Certain dietary considerations on unwell days can help prevent potentially serious problems of type 1 diabetes. Ensure that your child is taking in plenty of liquids, in most cases, It is best for your son or daughter to drink gradually rather than in large gulps. Tea, and undoubtedly, drinking water, are ideal options.

If your son or daughter struggles to eat a standard food, make sure they're taking in a degree of liquid or solid carbohydrates to avoid sudden drops in blood sugar. But always follow the precise recommendations from your wellbeing care professional.

Below are the right examples of drinks and foods for ill days:

- Sugar-containing drinks (sugar-free fluids may be consumed if blood sugar levels are raised)

- Fruit juice

- Sports drinks

- Jell-o

- Popsicles

- Broth-based soups

- Saltines

- Applesauce

- Bananas

- Toast

- Graham crackers

When to get Medical Attention there are a variety of situations that warrant medical assistance. If your son or daughter is having troubles breathing and/or has already established at least 3 shows of throwing up or diarrhea within an individual day, call your physician. Also, if huge amounts of ketones stay in your son or daughter's urine after a long time, seek medical assistance. Obviously, please call your wellbeing care professional.

CHAPTER 10

Meal Planning Children with Type 1 Diabetes

When you have a kid with type 1 diabetes, you can get overly enthusiastic with the idea of a diabetic diet. However, in reality, your son or daughter's nutritional needs are not the same as a kid who does not have diabetes. Obviously, there are specific considerations you should be alert to, in this specific article, become familiar with about the need for carb keeping track of, with a particular emphasis about how fiber and sugars alcohols could also affect your son or daughter's blood sugar (blood glucose) levels.

Nutrition Basics

That is why you should concentrate instead on providing

your son or daughter with balanced nourishment. A good dietary resource to seek advice from is the meals Pyramid. Lately, rather than being truly a set-in-stone guide, you will create personalized diet programs that are versatile and well balanced. Proteins, this essential nutrition affect blood sugar in various ways.

Fats: Body fat typically doesn't breakdown into sugars in your bloodstream, and in smaller amounts, it doesn't impact your blood sugar levels. But fats does decelerate digestion, your child's blood sugar may be raised up to 12 hours following the meal.

Proteins: Proteins doesn't affect blood sugar unless you eat even more than the body needs. Generally, you need no more than 6 oz. or less (which is approximately how big is 2 decks of credit cards) at each food.

Carbohydrates: Carbohydrates influence your blood sugar more than some other nutrient. All the sugars in food become glucose in the bloodstream, and they enter the bloodstream at a more speedily rate than fat and protein. Carbs usually enter the bloodstream one hour after intake and are usually from the bloodstream in 2 hours. That is why you should check your son or daughter's blood sugar levels before he or she eats, and on the other hand 2 hours later. Preferably, Whether it's not,

Carb Counting, Diet Plans, And Insulin Adjustment

For those who have type 1 diabetes, knowing the quantity of carbohydrates in the meals you eat is vital. Regrettably, your physician will determine the correct dose for your son or daughter.

It's simple enough to look for the total amount of sugars in the meals your son or daughter eats. All packed foods include a Nourishment Facts label, and which has the total sugars in each meal. If the meals does not have a label, your dietitian can provide you resources which contain the carbohydrate count number of common foods.

Everyone responds differently to sugars. He or she will establish a balanced food plan specifically for your son or daughter that is dependent on your son or daughter's food preferences, dietary needs, while others enable more versatility). The food plan will support the right amount of sugars for your son or daughter.

Rather, they help you select from specific food organizations. This can help you manage the quantity of sugars in each food, while still offering your son or daughter a balanced collection of food. Such as birthday celebrations.

For healthy development, it's important that your son or daughter follows his / her food plan. Not merely when your child eats from the meals groups defined in the program, but she or he also needs to eat them at a particular time. Eating foods and arranging insulin injections at exactly the same time every day aids in preventing blood sugar levels from getting away from control. Parents with youngsters could find this facet of type 1 diabetes management relatively easier than parents who've teenagers. Not merely are teenagers busier with activities and interpersonal schedules, however they are also transitioning to handling their diabetes with no help of their parents.

Fiber and the sort 1 Diabetes Diet

Found mainly in fruits, vegetables, coffee beans, and wholegrains, fiber may reduce bloodstream cholesterol, assist in weight reduction.

With regards to fitted fiber into your son or daughter's type 1 diabetes meal plan, you must understand how fiber impacts a food's true carbohydrate count. Luckily, it's a simple formula.

If the meals contains at least 5 grams of soluble fiber, simply subtract half the grams of fiber from the full total carbohydrate grams (you can certainly find these details on the Nourishment Facts label on packaged foods). The full total equals the web carbohydrate count number in the meals. For instance, if a food consists of 10 grams of total sugars and 5 grams of soluble fiber, the quantity of carbs that will have an effect on your child's blood sugar is 7.5 grams.

Soluble fiber may have less effect on blood sugar since it isn't soaked up 100% and releases glucose in to the cells more slowly. You can subtract the quantity of fiber from the full total carbohydrate. However, artificial types of fiber are being put into many processed food items, which might not supply the same advantage as natural foods.

A Special Notice about Sugars Alcohols

Foods with sugars alcohols (sorbitol) on the component list are favored by people who have diabetes. Such as candies, nibbling gums, contain glucose alcohols.

Unlike regular sugars, in addition they contain fewer calorie consumption than pure glucose.

Products made out of sugar alcohols tend to be geared toward people who have diabetes, when consumed in managed amounts, sugars alcohols won't result in blood glucose to go up. But if consumed in excess, the products will increase blood sugar in people who have type 1 diabetes. You'll want to understand that foods made out of glucose alcohols still contain sugars. Always ensure that you check the full total carbohydrates outlined on the Diet Facts. This can help you better learn how to fit them into your son or daughter's meal plan.

CHAPTER 11

Controlling Type 1 Diabetes at Classes

Type 1 diabetes requires continuous attention-it doesn't disappear completely during college hours. That is why it's essential that college staff, including educators, bus motorists, and college health staff.

A lot more than 13,000 teenagers are identified as having type 1 diabetes every year. it is important that colleges have at least some workers who have a simple knowledge of type 1 diabetes. Using a college worker readily available who understands how to check on blood sugar, inject insulin.

Resources for Parents and College Staff

That's a huge responsibility for parents and college

workers, but luckily, there are resources open to help make your son or daughter's college conducive to controlling type 1 diabetes.

Laws Protecting Your Son Or Daughter With Type 1 Diabetes

As a mother or father of a kid with type 1 diabetes, you ought to know of the federal government laws and regulations that protect your son or daughter at school. Here are short overviews of the laws. The explanations likewise incorporate links for connecting you to more descriptive information.

Section 504 of the Treatment Take action of 1973 and People in America with Disabilities Work of 1990 (ADA): Section 504 prohibits universities who receive government money from discriminating against people who have disabilities. Name II of the ADA prohibits institutions from discriminating against people who have disabilities, whether or not the institution receives federal money. Students with diabetes have always been included in both Section 504 and the ADA. For a far more extensive summary of these laws and regulations, go to the US Division of Education's Office for Civil Rights website.

"And also to be eligible, a child's diabetes must adversely impact their educational performance to the idea that he / she requires special education. To find out more,

Family Education Rights and Personal privacy Action (FERPA): FERPA prevents academic institutions from releasing any private information, including whether your son or daughter has diabetes, For more information, go to the US Section of Education's Family Plan Conformity Office website.

Also remember that specific says and individual school districts have laws and tips regarding a school's responsibility because of its students with type 1 diabetes. Visit your state's education website and/or contact your college district to find out more about the regulations that protect your son or daughter at college when he or she has type 1 diabetes. You can even contact your neighborhood ADA and JDRF offices to find out more.

CHAPTER 12

Hypoglycemia in Children with Type 1 Diabetes

Hypoglycemia, or low blood sugar, is a common problem that may appear with diabetes. First, it is critical to have a good knowledge of hypoglycemia. Endocrine Web has a thorough article series upon this complication-and we request you to learn them for more information. Below is an array of hypoglycemia resources to truly get you started:

- Hypoglycemia Overview

- Hypoglycemia Causes

- Hypoglycemia Treatment

  Detecting Hypoglycemia

Hypoglycemia occurs whenever your child's blood sugar levels fall below his / her target range.   1 Knowing your son or daughter's focus on range and making sure his / her blood sugar level remains within it is the primary objective.

If hypoglycemia isn't detected in early stages, such as seizure or lack of consciousness.

First and most important, you should comprehend the symptoms. Included in these are:

- Sweating

- Hunger

- Dizziness and difficulty concentrating

- Shakiness

- Headache

- Fatigue

- Pale skin

- Irritability

Ensure that you, your loved ones, as well as your child can identify the most typical hypoglycemia symptoms.

Treating Hypoglycemia

You should talk to your physician for specific suggestions on how to take care of your child if she or he experiences a bout of hypoglycemia. But, generally, if your son or daughter has a minimal blood sugar meter reading and it is displaying hypoglycemia symptoms, the target is to get your son or daughter's blood sugar level back to a wholesome range.

To get this done, blood sugar tablets, full-sugar (as with not diet) juice and carbonated drinks, and hard chocolate are good options. It might take 15-20 minutes for blood sugar to go up. If your son or daughter's blood sugar readings remain low after this time, give your son or daughter another providing of rapid performing carbohydrate.

So Prepare Yourself

Continually be prepared for the probability that your son or daughter may experience hypoglycemia. drinks, and blood sugar tablets. Ensure that your child has blood sugar tablets with her or him whatsoever times-during school, sports activities methods, extracurricular activities, and slumber celebrations.

When your son or daughter loses consciousness from severe hypoglycemia, demand emergency help and present your son or daughter an injection of glucagon-do not inject insulin. Glucagon is a hormone that creates the quick release of glucose into the bloodstream. Be sure you have multiple glucagon crisis kits-one for your home, car, as well as your child's school.

Nighttime Hypoglycemia

Regulating your son or daughter's blood sugar levels at

night time can be considered a tightrope walk, as they say. When blood sugar levels fall too low at night time, nighttime hypoglycemia might occur.

Nighttime hypoglycemia-or hypoglycemia occurring whenever your child is asleep-is seen as a night time sweats, headaches, and nightmares.

There are a variety of things that can trigger nighttime hypoglycemia. Increased exercise can make the insulin your son or daughter takes far better, meaning she or he might not need as much at foods and overnight.

With any change to your son or daughter's schedule, it's important that more blood sugar testing occurs, this can help identify how to modify the insulin to be able to reduce the chance of hypoglycemia.

The very best defense against hypoglycemia is diligent blood sugar monitoring to be able to recognize the way the many variables in your day affect your son or daughter's blood sugar level. However, the truth remains that children with type 1 diabetes-even people that have the most vigilant of parents-will likely experience hypoglycemia sooner or later. But if you understand the symptoms and are ready for the likelihood of a show, your child can make an instant recovery.

CHAPTER 13

Exercise For Children With Type 1 Diabetes

Children, have to be dynamic. Teaching the need for exercise in early stages will form healthy practices that will aid your son or daughter well into adulthood. But exercise also impacts blood sugar levels, so that as a parent, you should know how to react to these changes.

For those who have diabetes, being energetic offers a slew of important health advantages. These include reducing blood sugar levels and enhancing your body's capability to use insulin.

Essentially, exercise helps your son or daughter control his or her diabetes. And over time, this will certainly reduce the probability of your son or daughter experiencing certain health issues related to diabetes.

Activities For Your Son Or Daughter With Type 1 Diabetes

Being active is most appropriate if it is done frequently. That is why you should uncover what activities most interest your son or daughter. If your son or daughter actually enjoys the experience, then it greatly escalates the odds that he or she will continue steadily to participate.

If your son or daughter is thinking about sports, but don't be concerned if your son or daughter doesn't want to take part in a structured activity. Your son or daughter can be just like active within your own yard as on the sports activities field. Encourage your son or daughter to try out outside with friends, trip a bicycle, or walk your dog.

Also, take benefit of the countless opportunities you have every day to set an example for your son or daughter.

Take the stairways rather than the elevator. Then opt never to drive and walk with your son or daughter instead. Embark on a walk collectively after supper. Although they aren't extreme rounds of exercise, these activities can help form healthy behaviors that produce a difference.

The best goal is to really get your child moving. An excellent guideline to check out is that your son or daughter should get one hour of exercise in each day1. That may appear to be a great deal, but remember, it generally does not need to be strenuous activity.

Blood Sugar And Physical Exercise

Exercise can result in blood glucose to drop. If your son or daughter's blood sugar level falls too low, it can cause hypoglycemia.

Here are some methods for you to help lessen the result of exercise on your son or daughter's blood sugar level:

- Give your son or daughter extra carbohydrates, prior to the activity.

- Check your son or daughter's blood sugar level before, during, and following the activity.

- Prepare a package that contains snack foods, glucose tablets, juice, drinking water, and any medications that your physician recommends for your son or daughter to try practices and game titles.

- Make sure to check blood sugar more frequently following the activity and overnight to evaluate if insulin doses have to be adjusted.

- If your son or daughter is within organized sports, Show the trainer how to react if there are a problem related to your son or daughter's condition.

Also, if crisis occur. Your son or daughter should wear this bracelet all the time, not only during exercise and exercise.

Though there are precautions you will need to take, it is important that your son or daughter participates in regular exercise when she or he has type 1 diabetes. The huge benefits greatly outweigh the potential risks, so you shouldn't be scared to encourage your son or daughter to exercise and become physically energetic. With the correct preparation, your son or daughter can fully benefit from the same activities as almost every other child.

Acknowledgments

The Glory of this book success goes to God Almighty and my beautiful Family, Fans, Readers & well-wishers, Customers and Friends for their endless support and encouragements.